NUTRITION FOR BETTER HEALTH OVER 60

A Short Guide on How to
Eat Well and Stay Well for Seniors

BAZ THOMPSON

CONTENTS

BEFORE YOU START READING

As a special gift, I included a logbook and my book, **"Strength Training After 40"** (regularly priced at $16.97 on Amazon) and the best part is, you get access to all of them.

FREE

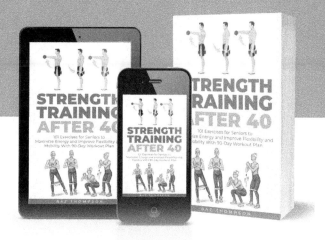

WHAT'S IN IT FOR ME?

- 101 highly effective strength training exercises that can help you reach the highest point of your fitness performance

- Foundational exercises to improve posture and increase range of motion in your arms, shoulders, chest, and back

- Stretches to help you gain flexibility and find deep relaxation

- Workout Logbook to help you keep track of your accomplishments and progress. Log your progress to give you the edge you need to accomplish your goals.

SCAN ME

INTRODUCTION

G ood nutrition is essential for good health. This is especially true for those over 60 years old. Because what we put into our bodies will form the building blocks for strong bones, lean muscle, and clear thinking, we want to pay attention to what we eat. As we grow older, how we fuel our bodies can help prevent and ward off common diseases and medical challenges.

This short book is specially designed for you, the reader over 60 years old. Eating well can help you to stay healthy as you move forward into your 70s, 80s, and beyond. If you are a caregiver, this book can be a good resource as you plan meals and snacks for your patient.

THE MALNUTRITION CRISIS

Nearly 50% of older adults risk being undernourished (Defeat Malnutrition Today, 2019). Are you as surprised as I am about this statistic? For many seniors, their bodies are not getting enough needed nutrients to function correctly. Malnourishment is a growing national concern in the United States because of its effect on health, well-being, and longevity.

According to a recent study, these are some effects of malnutrition in the older population (Norman et al., 2021):

- The annual cost of $53 billion for disease-related malnutrition
- Decrease in critical thinking and cognitive function
- Depression and anxiety
- Difficulty in recovering from colds, flu, and other diseases
- Fatigue and frailty
- Greater risk of falling
- Higher hospital admittance
- Impairment of the immune system and ability to fight infectious disease
- Increase in mortality rate
- Longer hospital stays
- Loss of bone density
- Loss of strength and mass in muscles
- More post-surgery complications

- Rise in inflammation
- Slower wound healing.
- Unwanted weight loss.

Being undernourished is not to be taken lightly. The consequences are real and have long-lasting effects.

What About You?

You might think that malnourishment occurs just in those who are underweight and sick. In fact, it can occur in anyone, even those who are overweight. It happens over several months to several years, so it can be hard to detect. There are several tools available online and at your doctor's office that can help you determine if you are undernourished. You can begin by asking yourself a few questions:

- Are my clothes looking looser on me?
- Do I eat less at each meal?
- Have I unintentionally lost weight in the last six months?
- Is my hand grip strength getting weaker?
- Am I more fatigued than usual?

These could be indicators of your body not getting the protein, vitamins, and minerals it needs. Lack of good nutrition—whether from a lack of food or eating the wrong foods—leads to malnourishment and its many repercussions.

Your doctor or healthcare provider is the best place to start if you suspect that you or a loved one are not getting the nutrients needed. A medical professional can screen and assess your current health status, make a correct diagnosis, and assist you in getting back on track.

HOW TO USE THIS BOOK

Now that we know more about malnutrition and how it affects people, we can move on to learning more about good nutrition, eating well, and staying healthy. This book is broken down into three easy-to-read, information-packed chapters.

Chapter 1 discusses why good nutrition can be a challenge and what obstacles present themselves. You may find that you have one, some, or several of these stumbling blocks in your life. We also talk about some ways to overcome these.

In Chapter 2, we look at the nutritional needs of older adults. You may already know some of the basics, but we delve into the specific food groups, how much you should eat, and how to work around certain dietary limitations and restrictions.

Healthy meal planning is covered in **Chapter 3**. Not only will you learn the best way to come up with a plan, but there is a sample five-day meal plan included for you!

Please check with your doctor or healthcare provider before making any changes or starting any new eating program. They know your particular health history and specific health concerns better than I do. Listen to their input and follow their guidelines. You can take this book with you to your next appointment to show them what you are learning and discuss how you plan to implement it.

My goal is to help you meet your nutritional needs by learning to overcome obstacles, identify what and how much you should be eating, and put together a game plan for weekly meals. You've already taken the first step by reading this far. So, let's get started!

CHAPTER 1
NUTRITION OBSTACLES AND SOLUTIONS

We know that good nutrition means eating the right foods in the right quantities. So what's the problem? The gap between knowledge and application is a challenge. You may know what you need to do, but for whatever reason, you don't or can't do it. You are not alone.

In this chapter, we look at some common reasons why older adults do not eat healthily and how these obstacles can be overcome. These challenges include allergies and dietary restrictions, dental problems, limited budget, medication side effects, mobility and physical challenges in preparing and eating food, and social isolation.

ALLERGIES AND DIETARY RESTRICTIONS

When you have food allergies or need to follow certain dietary restrictions for health or religious reasons, it can be a stumbling block to getting the right nutrients.

Ninety percent of allergic reactions to food come from the following items (U.S. Food and Drug Administration, 2021):

- Crustacean (shellfish)
- Eggs
- Fish
- Milk
- Peanuts
- Soybeans
- Tree nuts (almonds, pecans, walnuts)
- Wheat

True food allergies make themselves known by cramps, diarrhea, hives, rash, swelling, tingling, and wheezing, among other responses. Some people have life-threatening allergic responses that include anaphylactic shock and require immediate medical attention.

If you experience obvious symptoms, you know to stop eating that particular food item. But sometimes the allergic reaction is mild and you may not realize that your tummy ache or skin rash is associated with what you ate. The best way to find out if you actually have a food allergy is by consulting with your doctor or healthcare provider and getting tested.

Some people may have dietary restrictions because of diabetes, high blood pressure, or other medical conditions. Others may need to avoid certain foods because of their religious beliefs.

SOLUTION

Make a list. Write down all the foods that you need to avoid. You may have a mental list that you keep in your head, but having a written list helps remind you and whoever may be helping you with your meals that these are foods that you must avoid.

Now that you have a list, you can plan your meals and snacks more easily. There is always an alternative or substitution for the foods you are avoiding, and we will talk more about that in the next chapter.

DENTAL AND CHEWING PROBLEMS

As people age, they can be challenged with dental issues. Loose or cracked teeth, periodontal disease, TMJ (temporomandibular joint), or ill-fitting dentures can all make chewing food difficult. In addition to dental difficulties, many older adults have xerostomia, or dry mouth. Saliva production can decrease with the use of certain medications, making it harder to swallow. This poses a problem when needing to swallow food after chewing.

SOLUTION

In addition to practicing good oral hygiene, schedule regular checkups with your dentist or oral care provider. They will clean, treat, and give guidance on the best way to keep your teeth and gums healthy. If you have ongoing dental challenges, you will find it helpful to cut food into small pieces or opt for easy-to-chew proteins, like eggs, fish, tofu, and yogurt. Dentists can also provide simple remedies for your reduced production of saliva. Drinking water or other liquids with meals can also help.

LIMITED BUDGET

Some seniors live on a more limited budget than they did earlier in life. Retirement, lack of savings, or high medical bills can all affect the amount of disposable income that is available. Additionally, older adults may opt for packaged or already prepared foods which require less effort but are usually more expensive than single ingredient items. Almost 10% of those over 60 are considered food insecure because of financial reasons (Ziliak & Gundersen, 2021).

SOLUTION

There are many government programs available to assist seniors and those who qualify to receive benefits to help them buy the food they need. SNAP, or the Supplemental Nutrition Assistance Program (formerly known as food stamps), provides monthly funds to help seniors with their grocery budgets. Each state has different qualifying criteria, but most all of them provide an electronic prepaid card that allows users to purchase baked goods, canned goods, dairy products, fresh fruits, vegetables, meats and other proteins, and non-alcoholic beverages (Thomas, 2022).

MEDICATION AND SIDE EFFECTS

Many seniors need to take medicines for ongoing health conditions, for pain relief after surgery, or for other reasons. Medications, either prescribed or over-the-counter, can have many different side effects that impact a person's ability, desire, and willingness to eat. These can include things like

- Appetite suppression
- Bioavailability of essential nutrients in food
- Diarrhea
- Digestion issues
- Drug potency
- Dry mouth
- Gastrointestinal difficulties

- Nausea
- Olfactory disturbance and loss of sense of smell
- Slowed metabolism (Aðalbjörnsson & Ramel, 2021)

Some side effects are not serious and will go away or lessen over time. However, some are bothersome and affect your relationship with food and meals.

SOLUTION

Keep track of your symptoms by writing them down. It's easy to think you will remember, but a written record will help you when you mention it to your doctor. Talk to your healthcare provider and pharmacist about your symptoms and your concerns. They may be able to adjust the dosage, medicine, or frequency. Finding the best balance plus adjusting expectations can help.

MOBILITY AND PHYSICAL CHALLENGES

Physical issues like arthritis, joint pain, neuropathy, and muscle strength can impair your ability to prep and cook your own meals. Lessened grip strength and finger flexion may make it more difficult to open boxes and food packaging. Weak muscles and a reduced capability to stand, walk, or drive can prevent older adults from shopping for groceries and preparing food to feed themselves. Simple tasks like slicing an apple or opening a can of beans can be difficult for those with physical challenges. This can be a hindrance in the practice of good nutrition and food choices.

SOLUTION

Many grocery stores offer cut-up fruits and vegetables in serving-size portions in the produce section. The deli and meat counter can slice meats for you. Although you will pay a little more, these options may be worth it to you, especially if you are not able to cut things yourself. Now there are also grocery and restaurant delivery services like Instacart, food pantries, and Meals on Wheels that can bring groceries and a prepared meal, right to your front door. Many churches and religious organizations also provide nutritious meals for free to those in their community.

SOCIAL ISOLATION

As we get older, the likelihood of us living alone increases. Twenty-seven percent of those over 60 live by themselves (Ausubel, 2020). This means 14.7 million older adults live alone. The percentages rise as people get older, with nearly half of all people over 75 years old living by themselves. We all like to keep our independence and stay in our own homes, but this can lead to social isolation, loneliness, and sometimes depression. Many older people who live alone are not motivated to cook or prepare healthy and balanced meals for themselves. It's also easy to skip a meal if you have no one to eat with or talk to at mealtime. This can lead to undernourishment.

SOLUTION

This will take some creativity on your part! Think about how you can be around others at mealtime, whether that is by going to the local senior center or a nearby restaurant. When I used to work at a restaurant, "Dave" was a regular customer. He was in his 70s and would come in alone to dine each Wednesday for the daily special. All the waitstaff loved Dave, and he looked forward to visiting with us each week.

You can schedule a weekly lunch date with friends or join a group that meets regularly for meals. There will always be meals that you will wind up eating alone, but with a bit of forethought, you can balance that with meals that you can enjoy with other people.

Now that we have tackled some of the common obstacles to good nutrition and addressed how to overcome them, we will look at what comprises good nutrition and how to achieve it.

CHAPTER 2
NUTRITIONAL NEEDS FOR OLDER ADULTS

You may remember learning about the food groups when you were in grade school. Do you recall what they are? Some of the information has changed over time. We will be talking not only about the current recommended essential food groups that you should be consuming, but also touch on the quantity and caloric needs that you have as an older adult. Finally, we will address some of the special considerations for people who are dairy-free, gluten-free, vegetarian, or vegan.

BASIC FOOD GROUPS

The USDA (U.S. Department of Agriculture) has published dietary recommendations for the U.S. population since 1894. Their nutrition guides have been changed and updated over the years. One of the most recognizable guides was put together in 1992 as the first food pyramid. Featured food groups included dairy, fruit, grains, meats and beans, oils and sweets, and vegetables. The pyramid was divided into horizontal slabs that showed how much of each type of food should be consumed for optimal health. The USDA updated the pyramid in 2005, and then again in 2011.

The nutrition guide, now called MyPlate, currently consists of a meal plate divided into four sections: fruits, grains, proteins, and vegetables. A small circle next to the plate represents dairy. This visual makes it easy to measure how much of each food group you should be consuming.

- Fruits (10%) + vegetables (40%) = 50% of your plate
- Grains (30%) + proteins (20%) = 50% of your plate
- Dairy in limited amounts

Next, we will learn about each of these groups and some common food items in each.

FRUITS

Whether they are canned, fresh, frozen, or dried, fruits bring some natural sweetness to your life along with vitamins, good carbohydrates, and fiber. Fresh is always best, but canned, frozen, and dried fruits can be good alternatives as long as they do not have added sugar. Be sure to eat a variety of fruits. Some types are listed here, but there are many others:

- Berries: blackberries, cranberries, grapes, raspberries, strawberries
- Citrus: grapefruit, kumquats, lemons, limes, oranges, tangerines
- Rore: apples, pears
- Melons: cantaloupe, honeydew, watermelon
- Stone/pit: apricots, cherries, nectarines, peaches, plums
- Tropical: bananas, coconuts, dates, figs, guava, kiwi, mangoes, papaya, pineapple

GRAINS

Grains provide complex carbohydrates to our bodies, giving us energy and fiber. Foods that are made from barley, cornmeal, oats, rice, or wheat are considered part of the grains category. These grains are most often processed and refined so they can be made into bread, cereals, crackers, and pasta. Because the bran and outer germ have been removed (which contains many nutrients), the refined grains are enriched with additional vitamins.

When you consume whole grains, you are getting natural fiber, iron, and vitamin B. What is considered a whole grain?

- Barley

- Brown rice

- Buckwheat

- Dulgur

- Millet

- Oatmeal

- Popcorn

- Quinoa

- Whole-wheat bread, crackers, pasta

PROTEINS

Foods with protein provide our bodies with energy, but they also provide the building blocks for our muscles and tissues to grow and repair themselves. These building blocks, called amino acids, are not stored by our bodies, so it is important to eat some type of protein every day. It is nutrient-dense and supplies needed nutrients in small servings. Protein can come from many different sources, not just meat and poultry. Vegetarians and vegans can get their protein from plants and seeds.

Animal-based Proteins

- Dairy and eggs: cheese, eggs, milk, yogurt

- Fish and seafood: fish, shellfish

- Meats: beef, goat, lamb, pork, veal

- Poultry: chicken, duck, turkey

Plant-based Proteins

- Legumes: beans, lentils, peas, peanuts
- Nuts and nut butter: almonds, cashews, macadamia, pecans, pistachios, walnuts
- Seeds and seed butter: chia, flax, pumpkin, sesame, sunflower
- Soy products: tempeh, tofu

VEGETABLES

Vegetables come in every size, shape, and color. They bring vitamins and minerals into our diets while also providing needed fiber and complex carbohydrates. The USDA recommends that 40% of our plate should consist of vegetables! There are so many types to choose from, so that should keep us from getting bored. They can be eaten raw or cooked, depending on the type.

Some of the most common vegetables include the following:

- **Bulbs and flowers:** artichoke, asparagus, broccoli, cauliflower, garlic, onions, shallots
- **Fruits used as vegetables:** avocado, bell peppers, chili peppers, cucumbers, eggplant, okra, summer squash, tomato, winter squash
- **Leafy greens:** arugula, bok choy, Brussels sprouts, cabbage, chard, kale, lettuce, spinach
- **Pulses:** all beans, peas, lentils

- **Roots and tubers:** beets, carrots, parsnips, potatoes, radishes, sweet potatoes, turnips, yams
- **Stem:** celery, fennel, green onions, leek, rhubarb

CALORIE NEEDS

Now that you have an idea of the types of foods your body needs, we will look at how much you should be eating. Each person will have a different amount of calories needed. Why is that? Because your caloric intake is dependent on several factors, including your age, gender, and activity level.

According to the USDA Dietary Guidelines for those over 60, the recommended calorie intake should include nutrient-dense foods that limit added sugars and saturated fats (USDA, 2020). The general calorie guidelines are calculated by your level of activity. Those who are not physically active require fewer calories than those who are moderately active or lead an active lifestyle with regular exercise.

- Women: 1,600 to 2,200 calories
- Men: 2,000 to 2,600 calories

SERVING SIZE AND QUANTITY

So what do these calories look like when you sit down to eat a meal? It is easier to think about it in terms of serving size. When we talk about a serving size, it usually means a typical amount, such as one cup or eight ounces.

But not all serving sizes are the same! You must remember the density of the food you are eating. For example, one serving of fresh apple slices might equal one cup, but one serving of dehydrated apple chips would be half a cup. Dried apples are more compact than fresh ones. The same goes for raw versus cooked vegetables.

For 2,000 calories a day, these are the daily serving sizes and quantity of food you should be eating to make every bite count (USDA, 2020).

- Vegetables: 2 ½ cups

- Fruits: 2 cups

- Grains: 6 ounces (3 ounces whole grains, 3 ounces refined grains)

- Dairy: 3 cups

- Proteins: 5 ½ ounces

By varying the types of vegetables, fruits, grains, dairy, and protein you eat from day to day, you can be sure to not only get a variety of the nutrients you need but also keep from getting bored with eating the same things.

SPECIAL CONSIDERATIONS

What about those of you who must avoid certain foods? Many people can no longer tolerate certain foods as they age or have been instructed by their doctor to avoid particular things. In this section, we will talk about what to do if you are dairy-free, gluten-free, vegetarian, or vegan.

DAIRY-FREE

Dairy is any food that contains milk or milk products, such as the milk of cows, goats, sheep, and water buffalo. Typical dairy products are butter, cheese, ice cream, milk, and yogurt. Many older adults find it harder to process dairy products and may need to take supplements to help them digest these products or avoid them altogether.

Keep in mind that if you are not able to eat dairy made from cow's milk, you may be able to consume items made from the milk of other animals. A personal example: My cousin found that he could not have cheese made from cow's milk. But through trial and error, he discovered that goat cheese and sheep's milk cheeses did not bother him in the least. It is worth investigating other animal milk products.

If you are on a dairy-free diet, there are many alternative kinds of plant-based milk that are now available at grocery stores. Common ones such as almond, coconut, hemp, oat, or rice can easily be found in both refrigerated and shelf-stable sections. There are also cheese, ice creams, and yogurts made from plant-based kinds of milk in the refrigerated and freezer sections.

GLUTEN-FREE

Gluten is formed by barley, rye, or wheat flour being combined with water to form a dough. The proteins in these flours are activated and develop a webbed network that helps give baked goods lift and lightness. Gluten gives bread the pleasantly chewy texture and heady aroma that we all love. However, for those who have celiac disease or have a gluten intolerance, gluten can cause bloating, constipation, diarrhea, and other gastrointestinal issues. Celiac disease is fairly rare, occurring in about one percent of the U.S. population, but many people may be undiagnosed. The only way to know if you have celiac or gluten intolerance is by being screened and tested by your doctor or healthcare provider.

If you must be on a gluten-free diet, you will find that you have many options now at the store. Look for baked goods and different kinds of pasta made with alternative flour, like almond, coconut, corn, rice, or specially made gluten-free flour blends. Also, keep an eye on food labels of canned and packaged foods that may contain wheat or gluten.

VEGETARIAN AND VEGAN

Sometimes doctors will guide you to a vegetarian or vegan diet in an effort to lower your risk of cancer, diabetes, heart disease, high blood pressure, or other medical conditions. Whether you have been directed to eliminate meat from your diet by your doctor or have made a personal decision to do so, you can eat well and stay well on a vegetarian and vegan diet.

What's the difference between the two?

- Vegetarians are those who do not eat meat. There are many ways that people practice vegetarianism. Most vegetarians will eat eggs and dairy products, and some even include fish.

- Vegans are a subsection of vegetarians who avoid meat and all foods that come from animals. This includes eggs, dairy products, and honey. Veganism is also a lifestyle choice where people who practice it also avoid animal sourced products like beeswax, gelatins, leather, and other products made from animals.

The biggest concern for vegetarians and vegans nutritionally is receiving enough quality protein, vitamin B, calcium, and vitamin D for their bodies.

If you are on a vegetarian or vegan diet, you are able to get adequate protein and vitamins through eggs, dairy products, nuts and seeds, pulses (beans, lentils, peas), and whole grains. It is important to work with your doctor or nutritionist to ensure that you are getting the right amounts to nourish your body and stay healthy. They can guide you in the specific quantities of foods you need.

This chapter has helped us to get a handle on the food groups, calories needed, and special considerations for eating well and staying well. Now, let's put this knowledge into action!

CHAPTER 3
HEALTHY MEAL PLANNING

Here is where we get to have some fun! Healthy meal planning gives you the opportunity to choose, plan, and shop for what you eat. When we have a say in what we are eating, we are more likely to enjoy our meals. The steps to meal planning are easy to follow and will become a habit over time. Remember your specific nutritional needs and calories. At the end of this chapter is a sample five-day meal plan to get you going.

First, let's address why you should create a meal plan. Isn't it easier to just have an idea of what to eat and go from there? Not really. By nature, we are forgetful people. We forget what we have in our pantries, we forget what we've eaten today, and sometimes we even forget to eat! Some other benefits of meal planning are:

- **Saving money**. How many times do you wind up throwing out fresh fruits and vegetables because you bought them thinking you will eat them "someday?" Having a plan saves you money because you know when you will be eating them.

- **Saving time.** How much time do you waste thinking about what you are going to make for dinner that night or wandering around a grocery store deciding what to buy? Having a plan gives you a clear list of items to buy while shopping and an idea of what to eat each day.

- **Including variety.** Do you wind up eating the same vegetables again and again? When you plan your meals, you also get to plan a variety. You can include different fruits, vegetables, grains, and proteins from week to week. Variety keeps things interesting at mealtime and provides you with different nutrients and micronutrients.

STEPS TO CREATING A MEAL PLAN

1. Look at your calendar and see what you have going on this coming week. Mark the days that you know you will be eating at home.

2. Think about what you'd like to eat. Maybe there is a certain cultural holiday or special day that you know you will want to have certain foods.

3. Write down your meal ideas and plan for leftovers. For instance, if you know you are having a meal with chicken and vegetables on Monday, you may have leftovers to use for Tuesday's lunch or dinner.

4. Take stock of what you already have in your fridge, freezer, and pantry. You may already have several ingredients you need.

5. Make a grocery shopping list. Be sure to include fresh, frozen, and shelf-stable items.

SAMPLE 5-DAY MEAL PLAN

Now that you know how to come up with a meal plan, we can look at a sample plan that can give you ideas. This plan is for five days of meals at home, which allows for two days that you may be dining out or enjoying a meal with friends.

Because the specific quantities that you will be eating are dependent on your size and calorie needs, we have not designated the serving size.

DAY 1

Breakfast: omelet with spinach and mushrooms, and a slice of whole-grain toast.

Lunch: chicken salad with cashews and grapes on lettuce

Snack: celery with peanut butter

Dinner: curried lentil soup

DAY 2

Breakfast: chocolate banana smoothie made with yogurt

Lunch: leftover curried lentil soup or egg salad sandwich on whole-grain toast

Snack: baby carrots with hummus

Dinner: baked salmon with asparagus

DAY 3

Breakfast: breakfast burrito of eggs, sausage, and avocado wrapped in a tortilla

Lunch: mini-charcuterie plate of deli turkey, cheese slices, pickles, olives, and berries

Snack: apple slices with almond butter

Dinner: vegetable lasagna, green salad

DAY 4

Breakfast: steel-cut oatmeal with fresh blueberries and chopped walnuts

Lunch: leftover veggie lasagna or tuna salad sandwich on whole-grain bread

Snack: cucumber slices with yogurt-dill dip

Dinner: beef stew with carrots, peas, and potatoes

DAY 5

Breakfast: strawberry spinach smoothie made with yogurt

Lunch: whole grain toast with mashed avocado, smoked salmon, and sliced onion

Snack: grapes and string cheese

Dinner: teriyaki chicken breast with broccoli and rice

CONCLUSION

You made it! Here we are at the end of this information-packed book about nutrition for older adults. I know that you have learned a lot on this journey. Whether you have read for yourself or for someone that you are caring for, this book has given you some practical information that you can build upon.

There is a growing concern about malnutrition and its effects on the aging population. You have learned that eating well and staying well is not only important for avoiding disease and illness, but it also benefits you financially by keeping you from prolonged hospital stays and medication costs. Good nutrition is also important for us physically and psychologically. Our brain and overall mood have much to gain from the nutrients we are putting into our bodies.

We've covered a lot in this book. It may help you to re-read it or revisit certain chapters from time to time.

In Chapter 1, we looked at some of the common challenges and obstacles to receiving good nutrition, such as allergies and dietary restrictions, dental problems, limited budget, medication side effects, mobility and physical challenges in preparing and eating food, and social isolation. We also covered the solution to overcoming these potential roadblocks.

Chapter 2 focused on the nutritional needs of older adults. It's important to know the basic food groups and know how much to eat in terms of calories and quantity. While there are some special considerations for those with specific dietary needs like dairy-free, gluten-free, vegetarianism, or veganism, we learned that good nutrition can still be achieved.

Healthy meal planning was covered in Chapter 3 and you got to see the easy-to-follow steps on how that can be done. With practice and time, meal planning will become a habit and something you can have fun with. To get you started, a sample five-day meal plan was outlined for you to follow.

Now that we are at the end of the book, how are you going to apply what you have learned? My hope and prayer are that you will continue learning and growing in your nutritional knowledge and application. Good nutrition is a choice and one that you will never regret making. Please consider leaving a review if you have found this book helpful. We would love to hear about how it has impacted and helped you!

SCAN THE QR CODE TO LEAVE A REVIEW:

I hope you enjoy good health and happiness on the long road ahead of you, and I wish you all the best. Thank you for allowing me to share my knowledge with you.

Baz Thompson

REFERENCES

Aðalbjörnsson, B. V., & Ramel, A. (2021). Food-drug Interaction in older adults. Perspectives in Nursing Management and Care for Older Adults, 249–259. https://doi.org/10.1007/978-3-030-63892-4_20

Ausubel, J. (2020, March 10). Older people are more likely to live alone in the U.S. than elsewhere in the world. Pew Research Center. https://www.pewresearch.org/fact-tank/2020/03/10/older-people-are-more-likely-to-live-alone-in-the-u-s-than-elsewhere-in-the-world/

Care Giver Asia. (2020, August 12). The top 5 nutritional problems that seniors commonly face. Blog.caregiverasia.com. https://blog.caregiverasia.com/the-top-5-nutritional-problems-that-seniors-commonly-face

Defeat Malnutrition Today. (2019). Focusing on malnutrition in healthcare helps. https://www.defeatmalnutrition.today/sites/default/files/images/DMT_Malnutrition_Info_Graphic_OnePage_Update_2.pdf

Kaplan, D., & Berkman, B. (2022, September). Older adults living alone - geriatrics. Merck Manuals Professional Edition. https://www.merckmanuals.com/professional/geriatrics/social-issues-in-older-adults/older-adults-living-alone

Mann, D. (2005, September 23). Eating right with limited mobility. WebMD. https://www.webmd.com/arthritis/features/eating-right-with-limited-mobility

MedlinePlus. (2019). Nutrition for older adults. Medlineplus. gov; National Library of Medicine. https://medlineplus.gov/nutritionforolderadults.html

National Institute on Aging. (2021, November 23). Healthy meal planning: Tips for older adults. National Institute on Aging. https://www.nia.nih.gov/health/healthy-meal-planning-tips-older-adults#:~:text=Choose%20foods%20with%20little%20to

National Institute on Aging. (2022a, February 25). Healthy eating as you age: Know your food groups. National Institute on Aging. https://www.nia.nih.gov/health/healthy-eating-you-age-know-your-food-groups

National Institute on Aging. (2022b, February 28). How much should I eat? Quantity and quality. National Institute on Aging. https://www.nia.nih.gov/health/how-much-should-i-eat-quantity-and-quality

National Institute on Aging. (2022c, April 7). Overcoming roadblocks to healthy eating. National Institute on Aging. https://www.nia.nih.gov/health/overcoming-roadblocks-healthy-eating

Norman, K., Haß, U., & Pirlich, M. (2021). Malnutrition in older adults—recent advances and remaining challenges. Nutrients, 13(8), 2764. https://doi.org/10.3390/nu13082764

Thomas, J. (2022, October 18). What is SNAP and I do I apply? Www.ncoa.org; National Council on Aging. https://www.ncoa.org/article/what-is-snap-and-how-do-i-apply

U.S. Department of Agriculture Food and Nutrition Service. (n.d.). Sample meal patterns for the healthy US-style food pattern at the 2000 calorie level. Retrieved November 29, 2022,

from https://fns-prod.azureedge.us/sites/default/files/usda_
food_patterns/SampleMealPatternsForTheHealthyUS-Style-
FoodPatternAtThe2000KcalLevel.pdf

U.S. Food and Drug Administration. (2021). Food allergies:
What you need to know. FDA. https://www.fda.gov/food/buy-
store-serve-safe-food/food-allergies-what-you-need-know

USDA. (2020). Dietary guidelines for Americans 2020 -2025
make every bite count with the dietary guidelines. https://
www.dietaryguidelines.gov/sites/default/files/2020-12/Di-
etary_Guidelines_for_Americans_2020-2025.pdf

Vranešić Bender, D., & Krznarić, Ž. (2020). Nutritional issues and considerations in the elderly: an update. Croatian
Medical Journal, 61(2), 180–183. https://doi.org/10.3325/
cmj.2020.61.180

Ziliak, J., & Gundersen, C. (2021). The state of senior hunger
in America in 2019. https://www.feedingamerica.org/sites/de-
fault/files/2021-08/2021%20-%20State%20of%20Senior%20
Hunger%20in%202019.pdf

Printed in the USA
CPSIA information can be obtained
at www.ICGtesting.com
LVHW021726021024
792743LV00003B/446